Asma Mensi
Emna Bel Hadj Mabrouk
Nouha Trad

Association between nutritional factors and hemorrhoids

Asma Mensi
Emna Bel Hadj Mabrouk
Nouha Trad

Association between nutritional factors and hemorrhoids

ScienciaScripts

Imprint

Any brand names and product names mentioned in this book are subject to trademark, brand or patent protection and are trademarks or registered trademarks of their respective holders. The use of brand names, product names, common names, trade names, product descriptions etc. even without a particular marking in this work is in no way to be construed to mean that such names may be regarded as unrestricted in respect of trademark and brand protection legislation and could thus be used by anyone.

Cover image: www.ingimage.com

This book is a translation from the original published under ISBN 978-620-6-71685-3.

Publisher:
Sciencia Scripts
is a trademark of
Dodo Books Indian Ocean Ltd. and OmniScriptum S.R.L publishing group

120 High Road, East Finchley, London, N2 9ED, United Kingdom
Str. Armeneasca 28/1, office 1, Chisinau MD-2012, Republic of Moldova, Europe
Printed at: see last page
ISBN: 978-620-7-90088-6

TABLE OF CONTENTS

INTRODUCTION

Haemorrhoidal disease is a common condition affecting many people. It affects around 40% of the general adult population. It can affect people of all ages, sexes and backgrounds. Haemorrhoidal disease is benign but can affect quality of life [1].Haemorrhoids are physiological anatomical structures normally present in healthy individuals. They are made up of venous lakes, small arterioles and an anastomotic network. They are organised into an internal haemorrhoidal plexus (above the pectineal line) and an external haemorrhoidal plexus (below the pectineal line, subcutaneous in the radial folds of the anus) (Figure 1).

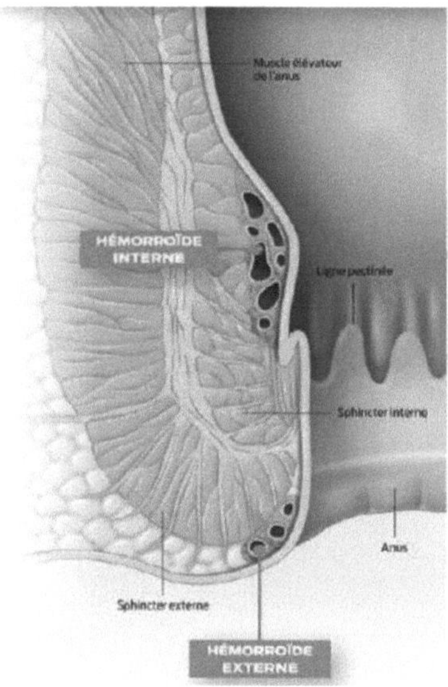

Figure 1:Representation of internal and external haemorrhoids

Haemorrhoidal disease is defined as all the symptoms associated with haemorrhoids. Internal haemorrhoidal disease must be distinguished from external haemorrhoidal disease, which are anatomically, pathophysiologically, clinically and therapeutically distinct entities [2,3]. The main symptoms of this condition are anal pain, rectal discharge and prolapse. haemorrhoids, itching... A number of risk factors are involved in haemorrhoidal disease, in particular age, hereditary factors, pregnancy, childbirth, the post-partum period, constipation with flare-ups, a sedentary lifestyle and alcohol [4,5]. Nutritional factors also play an important role in this frequent proctological pathology [6]. However, the literature on the association between diet and haemorrhoids is limited.The primary objective of this study was to identify the main dietary habits associated with haemorrhoidal disease. Our secondary objectives were to investigate the epidemiological and clinical factors associated with this disease.

METHODOLOGY

1. Type, location and duration of study :

This is a cross-sectional comparative descriptive study conducted in the gastroenterology department of the Charles Nicolle Hospital over a period running from 20/11/2023 to 15/12/2023 and from 15/01/2024 to 02/02/2024.

2. Study population :

2.1. Inclusion criteria: We included 2 groups of patients:

2.1.1. Group 1: Patients followed up at the gastroenterology outpatient clinic for haemorrhoidal disease.

2.1.2. Group 2: control group. In this group, we included volunteer patients who were being monitored for other conditions and who did not have haemorrhoidal disease.

2.2. Non inclusion criteria

- Under 18 years of age.

- Other proctological pathologies: anal margin abscess, anal fistula, etc.

- Colorectal cancer

2.3. Exclusion criteria :

Patients who did not cooperate with t h e questioning and investigation were excluded from this study.

food.

3. the study

3.1. Data collection: Data collection was based on questioning. We

collected the following parameters for each patient:

- Full name

- Age, gender

- Civil status

- Level of education, profession

- Socio-economic conditions

- Geographical origin

- Physical activity level (PAL): The PAL was estimated using a questionnaire including questions on physical activity during leisure time [7].
Physical activity was defined as :

1. **Sedentary**: almost no activity at all

2. **Light**: for example, walking, cycling or light gardening about once a week.

3. **Moderate**: regular activity at least once a week, such as walking, cycling or gardening, or walking to work for 10 to 30 minutes a day.

4. **Active:** regular activities more than once a week, such as brisk walking, cycling or playing sports.

5. **Very active:** intense activity several times a week

- Personal and family history of diabetes, hypertension, obesity or other pathologies.
- Gynaecological and obstetric history in women

3.2. Lifestyle :

- Smoking

- Alcoholism

3.3. Functional signs :

- We looked for transit problems such as diarrhoea or constipation.

➢ Diarrhoea is defined as stools that are too heavy (stool weight > 300g/day) and/or too frequent (> 3 stools/day) and/or too liquid (water weight greater than 90% of stool weight).
➢ Constipation is defined as infrequent bowel movements (< 3 bowel movements/week) or dissatisfaction during defecation or difficulty in exonerating.
➢ Defecation effort

- Anal pain, its intensity, onset and evolution...

- Rectorrhagia, defined as the discharge of bright red, undigested blood from the anus.

- Anal pruritus...

3.4.Physical examination :

Anthropometric measurements were collected:

- Weight (kg)

- Height (m)

- Body mass index (BMI) :

Which is used to classify the nutritional status of patients according to theWHO classification [8]. It is calculated according to the following formula:

BMI: weight/height^2 (kg/m^2)
Table I: WHO BMI classification

Classification	BMI (kg/m^2)	Risks
Severe malnutrition	<17	
Leanness	<18.5	
Normal	18.5 - 24.9	
Overweight	25 - 29.9	Moderately increased
Grade I obesity	30 - 34.9	Moderate or severe obesity commune
Grade II obesity	35 - 39.9	Severe obesity
Grade III obesity	> 40	Massive or morbid obesity

BMI: body mass index

- Waist circumference (WC) (cm): was measured using a tape measure placed midway between the anterior superior iliac spine and the costal margin, parallel to the ground. The measurement w a s taken at the end of exhalation.

Abdominal obesity has been defined according to the WHO [9] :
- **In women:** TT $\geq$ 80 cm

- **In men:** TT $\geq$ 94 cm

3.5. The proctological examination :

It is performed in the pectoralis genius position and comprises 2 stages:
- Inspection of the anal margin to look for spontaneous haemorrhoidal prolapse or haemorrhoidal prolapse caused by pushing, haemorrhoidal thrombosis in the form of a painful, tense, bluish swelling at the anal margin (figure 2), or an associated anal fissure.

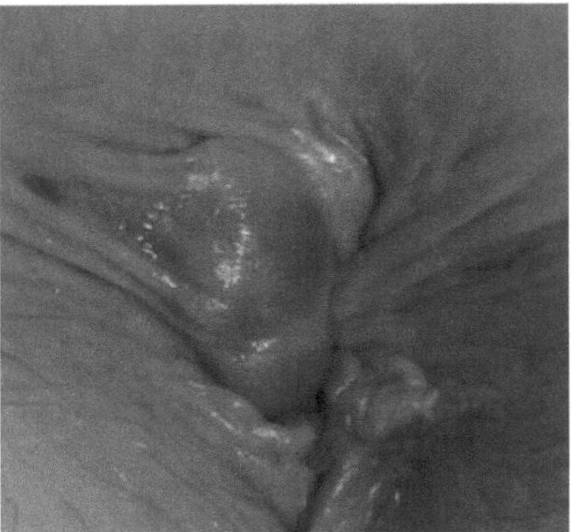

Figure 2:Haemorrhoidal thrombosis

- Anoscopy: used to explore the anal mucosa (figure 3).

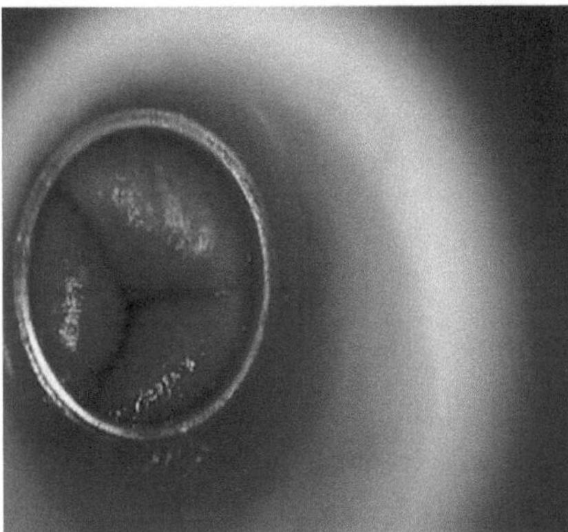

Figure 3: Anoscopic view of internal haemorrhoids

On completion of this examination, the haemorrhoids are classified into 4 stages according to the Goligher classification [10] :

Table II: The different grades of internal haemorrhoids

Grade I	Non-prolapsed congestive haemorrhoids.
Grade II	Haemorrhoids prolapsing during defecation (or during exertion) and spontaneously reintegrating after passing stool.
	Haemorrhoids prolapsing during defecation (or during exertion) and requiring manual reintegration
Grade IV	Permanently prolapsed haemorrhoids that cannot reintegrate manually.

3.6. Biological work-up :

We collected blood count data, in particular haemoglobin levels, to assess the impact of haemorrhoids.

3.7. Colonoscopy :

Allows you to visualise internal haemorrhoids and, above all, to rule out another cause of haemorrhoids. rectorrhagia, particularly colorectal cancer.

3.8. Food survey :

The survey was used to assess dietary habits, in particular:
- Tobacco and alcohol

- Average water consumption

- Consumption of salty foods (table salt, salted snacks, ready-made meals, canned soups, ready-made sauces, etc.),
- Consumption of spicy foods (paprika, pepper, chilli peppers....),

- Consumption of strong condiments (pickled vegetables, vinegar, hot sauces, hot oils, mustard, etc.),

- Average consumption of caffeinated drinks: coffee and tea,

- Cooking methods, snacking, skipping meals

During the food survey, we defined:

- Low consumption: Rarely or never

- Moderate consumption: one to three times a week

- Consumption High: more than three times a week Types of surveys used :
- a frequency survey: frequency of consumption of various foods (fruit,
vegetables, meat, wholegrain cereals.....)

- a nutritional survey such as a food history :

Quantification was estimated using household measurements (bowl, cup, glass,
ladle, soup spoon, teaspoon) and using Ms Bouchoucha's manual on Tunisian
foods (appendix).The results of the dietary survey were then processed by
appropriate software, NUTRILOG online, based on the CIQUAL 2020
composition table validated and made available by ANSES (the French food
safety agency), in order to make a general assessment of the patients' nutritional
status.To sum up, we essentially studied the following elements:

- Total calorie intake (Kcal)

- Carbohydrate composition of the diet (%) (g)

- Protein composition of the diet (%) (g)

- Fat composition of the diet (%) (g)

- Composition of fibre in the diet (g)

3.9. Statistical study :

The data were first entered using Excel 2013 and then analysed using SPSS
version 27.

- For the descriptive study :

For quantitative variables, means, extremes and standard deviations were
calculated. For qualitative variables, frequencies and percentages were
calculated.
- For the comparative study :
The Chi^2 test is used to study the independence between two qualitative
variables
The ANOVA test is used to study the effect of a qualitative variable known as a

factor.on a quantitative variable

- The decision rule for these tests depends on the value of the result p with a significance level of 5% (0.05) :

If p>0.05, there is no statistically significant relationship and the two variables are independent,

If p<0.05, there is a statistically significant relationship (link and dependency) between the two variables.

3.10.Ethical considerations :

For each patient, we explained the course and aims of the study, and we took his or her name.consent.Data was entered and processed anonymously.

1. Descriptive study :

1.1.Demographics of the patient population :

We included 30 patients

1.1.1. Genre :

The sex ratio (female/male) of our population was 1.72 (Figure 4).

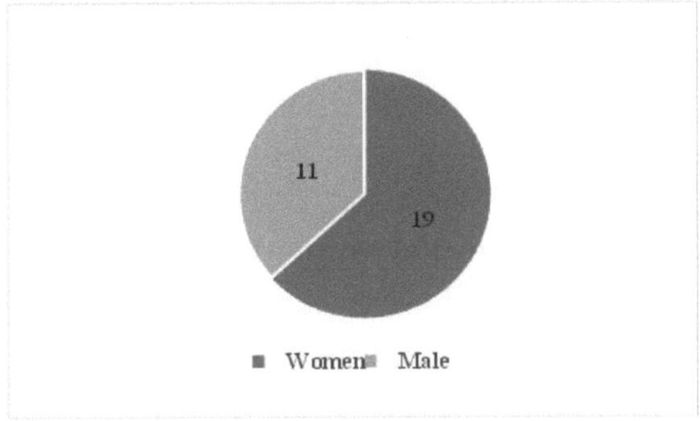

Figure 4: Breakdown of patients by gender

1.1.2. Age :

The average age of patients was 46.2 ± 14.4 years, with extremes ranging from 21 to 67 years. The 50-59 age group accounted for 27% of the population. The other age groups are shown in Figure 5.

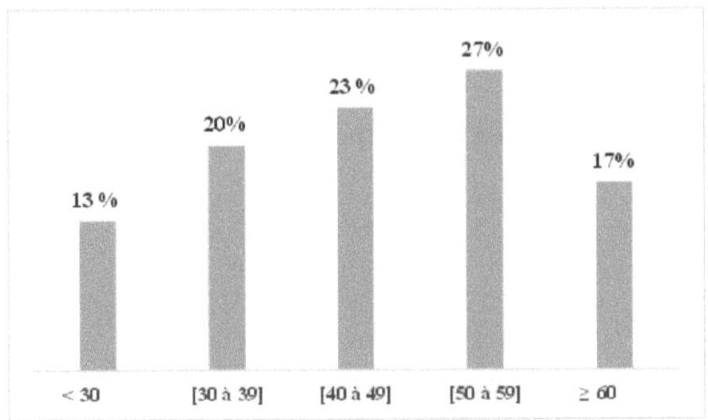

Figure 5: Breakdown of patients by age

1.1.3. Level of education :

Higher level patients represented the largest category of the order of 37%. Illiteracy accounted for 10% of patients. (Figure 6).

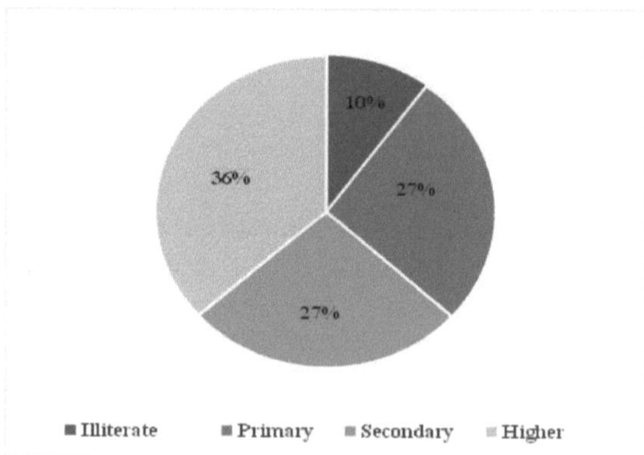

Figure 6: Distribution of patients by level of education

1.1.4. Marital status :

Seventy per cent of our patients were married (Figure 7).

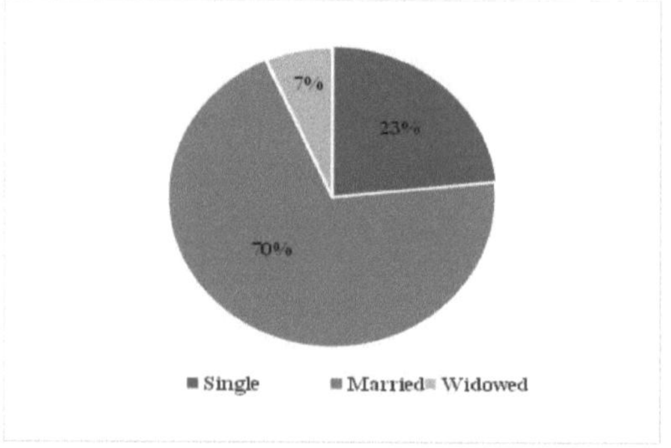

Figure 7:Distribution of patients by marital status

1.1.5. Socio-economic status :

More than half the patients (67%) had an average socio-economic status. (Figure 8).

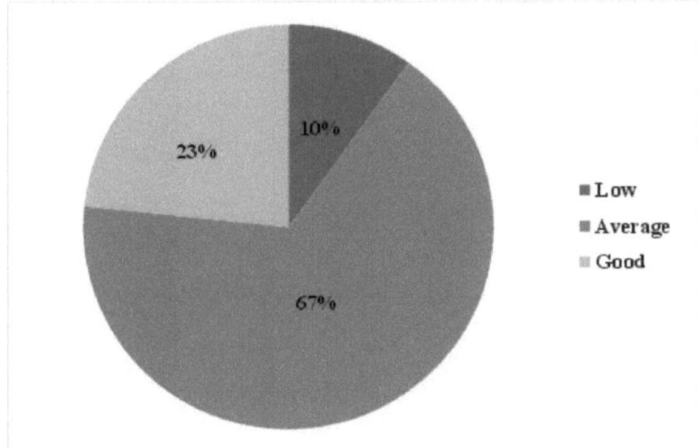

Figure 8: Breakdown of patients by socio-economic status

1.1.6. Geographical origin :

The majority of patients were from urban areas (93%).

1.1.7. Personal history :

Our study concluded that 4 patients were obese, 4 patients had diabetes and 8 patients had hypertension.

1.1.8. Family history :

Diabetes (60%) and hypertension (46.7%) were the pathologies most frequently found in the family histories of our patients. (Figure 9).

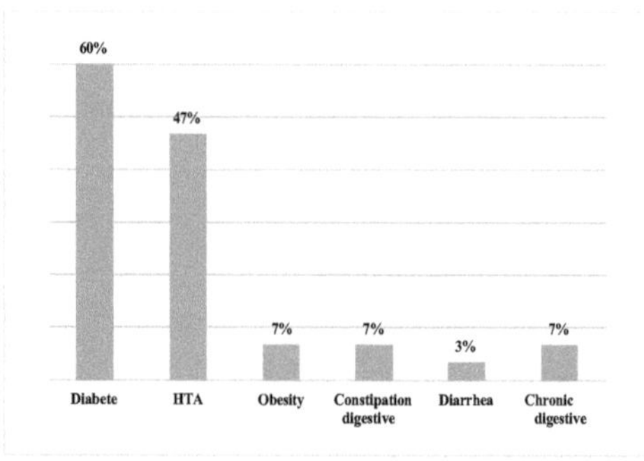

Figure 9: Distribution of patients according to family history

1.1.9. Gynaeco-obstetric history in women :

Most women with haemorrhoids had a history of pregnancy (Figure 10).

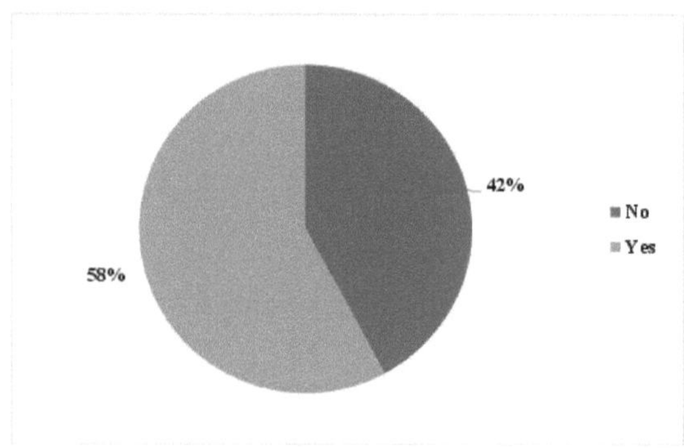

Figure 10: Distribution of patients by pregnancy history

1.1.10. Level of physical activity :

The majority of our patients were sedentary or had a low level of physical activity (Figure 11).

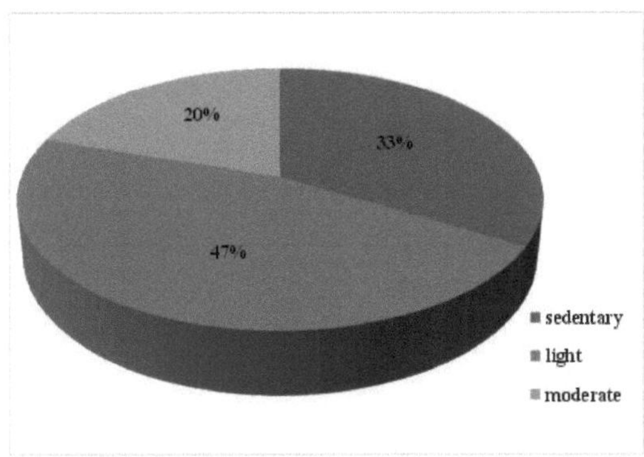

Figure 11: Distribution of patients by level of physical activity

1.2. Anthropometric measurements :

The average weight of the patients was 74.6 ± 18.34 kg, with extremes ranging from 46.5 to 121 kg. The mean BMI was 26.99 ± 5.86 kg/m² with extremes ranging from 17.9 to 43.9 kg/m². The other measurements are shown in the table below (Table III)

Table III: Anthropometric measurements of patients

	Average	Standard deviation	Minimum	Maximum
weight/kg	74,16	18,34	46,5	121,0
size/cm	148,11	50,56	1,65	186,00
BMI	26,99	5,86	17,90	43,90
waist circumference	88,12	9,79	67,0	109,0

BMI: body mass index

The distribution of patients by BMI is shown in Figure 12 below.

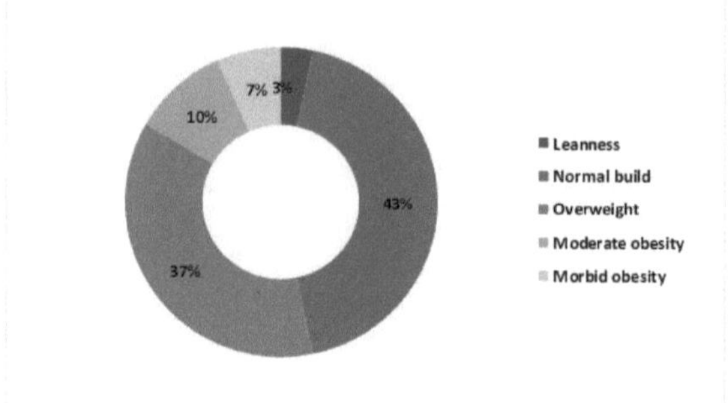

Figure 12: Distribution of patients according to BMI

1.3. Functional signs :

With regard to functional signs, most patients presented with constipation (77%). Jaundice was present in 63%. (Figure 13)

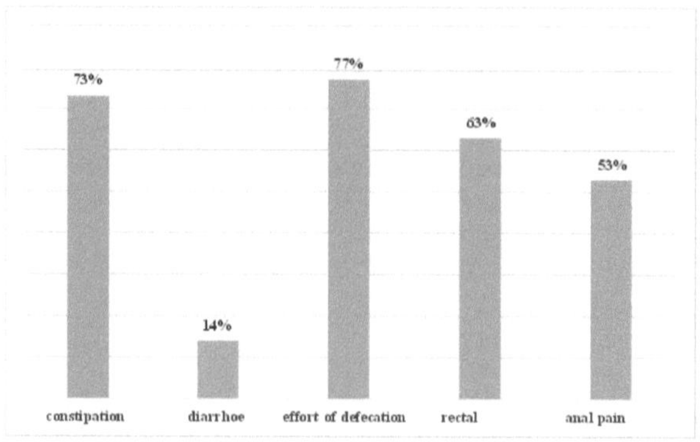

Figure 13: Distribution of patients according to functional signs

- Onset of illness :

The functional signs associated with haemorrhoids (anal pain, rectal discharge) had been present for one week in 8 patients, for 1 month in 4 others, for 6 months in 6 patients and for more than a year in the last 6 patients.

- Onset of the disease in women following pregnancy:

Haemorrhoidal disease was discovered during pregnancy in 1/3 of patients.

- Classification of haemorrhoids :

Internal haemorrhoids were the most common in our patients (Figure 14).

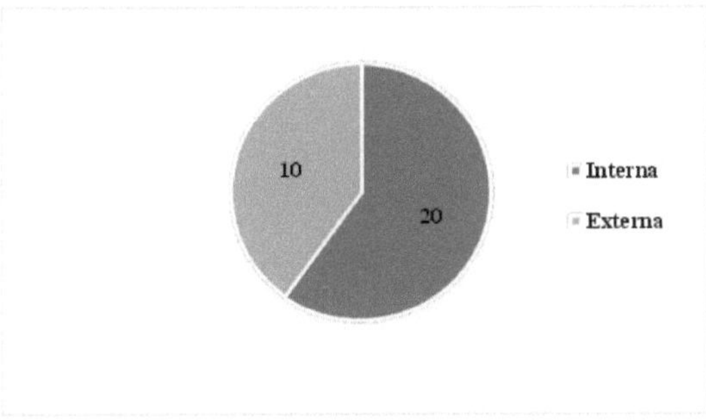

Figure 14: Distribution of patients by type of haemorrhoid

- Grades of internal haemorrhoids:

Most patients with internal haemorrhoids were grade 2, as shown in Figure 15.

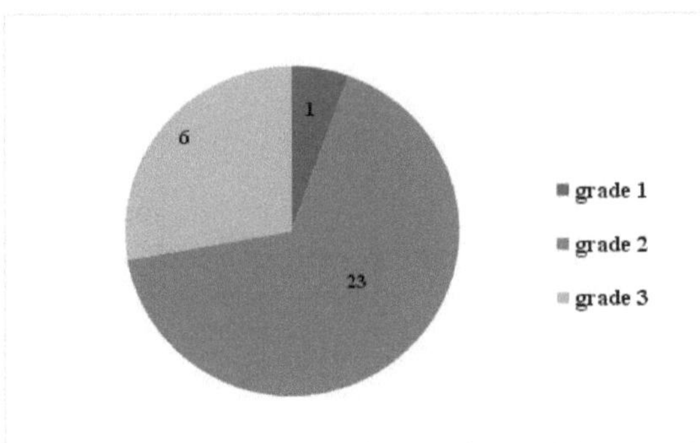

Figure 15: Distribution of patients according to haemorrhoid grade

- The presence of haemorrhoidal thrombosis :

Seventeen patients had haemorrhoidal thrombosis. These were mainly external haemorrhoids (10 patients had external haemorrhoids and 7 patients had internal haemorrhoids).

1.4. Biological check-up :

1.4.1. Haemoglobin level :

Microcytic hypochromic anaemia was observed in 60% of patients (Figure 16).

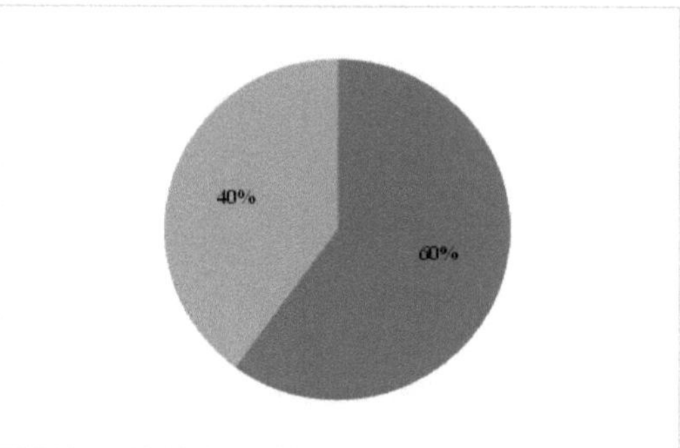

Figure 16: Distribution of patients according to the presence of anaemia

1.5. Data from colonoscopy :

Most patients (23) underwent colonoscopy. It was normal except for haemorrhoids in all these patients.

1.6. The current treatment :

Most patients were treated locally (47%). Venotonic therapy was prescribed in 30% of cases. Treatment of constipation was prescribed in ¾ of patients.

2. Comparative study :

2.1. Comparison of demographic characteristics :

2.1.1. Gender comparison :

The 2 groups were comparable with regard to gender (p=0.791) as shown in the figure below. (Figure 17)

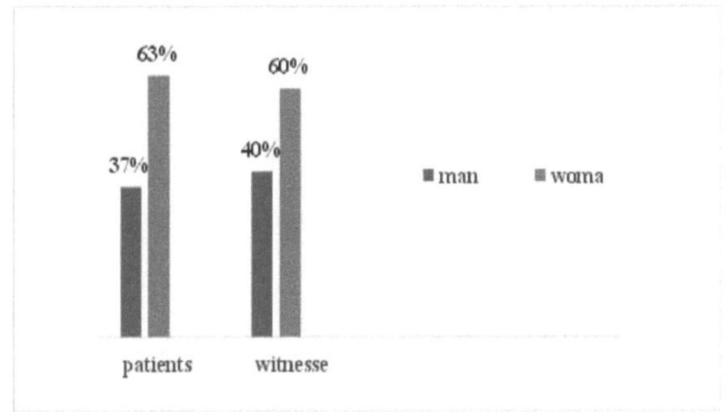

Figure 17: Breakdown of the two groups by gender

2.1.2. Comparison by age :

The mean age of subjects in the control group was 44.5 ± 19.8 years, and was comparable with that in the patient group (p =0.069) (Figure 18).

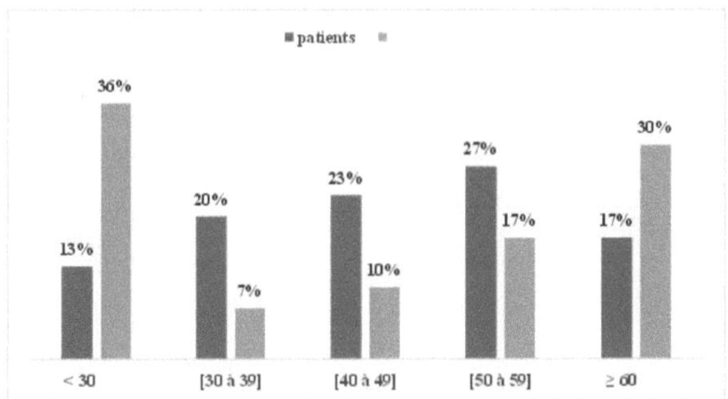

Figure 18: Breakdown of population by age group

2.1.3. Comparison by personal history :

In terms of pathological history, the two groups were comparable (p=0.484) (Figure 19).

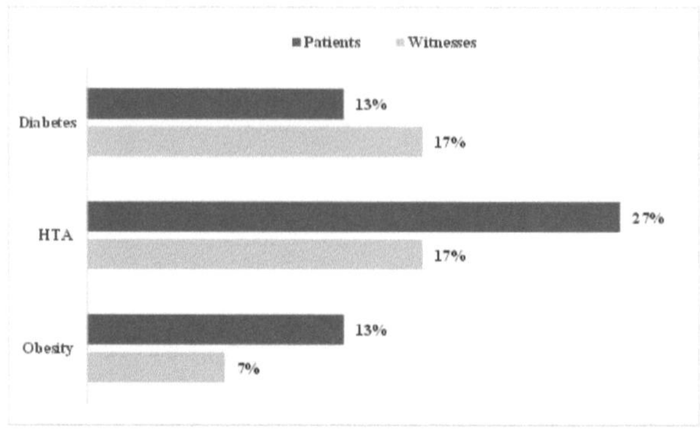

Figure 19: Breakdown of groups by medical history

Our study showed that 43% of patients and 13% of controls had chronic constipation, with a significant difference (**p = 0.01**) (Figure 20).

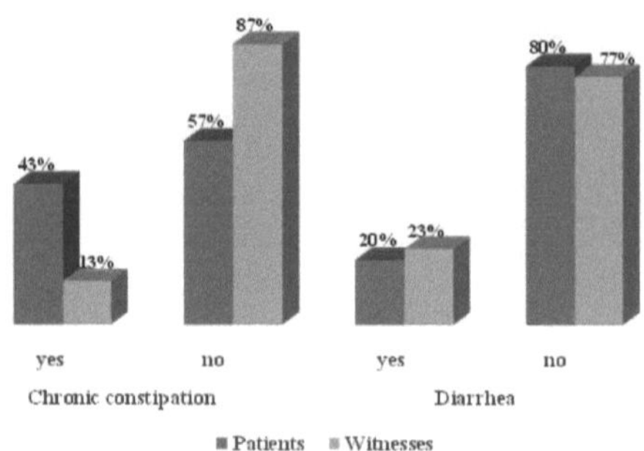

Figure 20: Comparison of groups according to transit disorders

2.1.4. Comparison by level of physical activity :

In the patient group, 33% of patients were sedentary, compared with 37% in the control group. The difference in NAP between the 2 groups was not statistically significant (p =0.518). The distribution of the groups according to the level of physical activity is shown in figure 21.

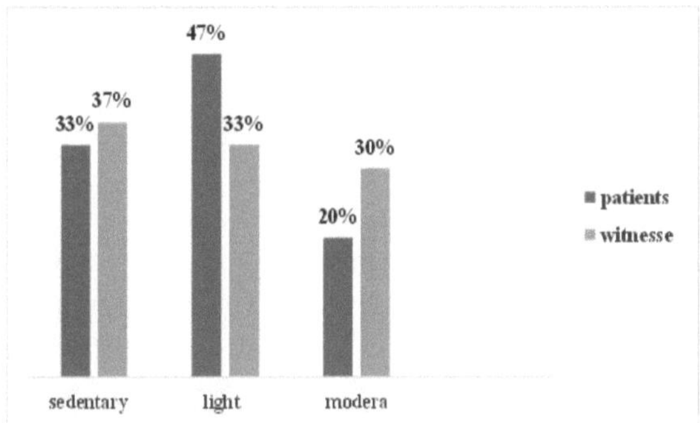

Figure 21: Breakdown of groups by level of physical activity

2.2. Comparison by weight and BMI :

The differences between the patient group and the control group were statistically significant. for weight and BMI (p = 0.001) (Table IV)

Table IV:Comparison of the two groups according to weight and BMI

	Patients			Witnesses			P
	Mean ± SD	Min	Max	Mean ± SD	Min	Max	
Weight (kg)	74,16 ± 18,34	46,5	121,0	59,72 ± 14,08	40,0	89,5	0,001
BMI (kg/m²)	26,99 ± 5,86	17,90	43,90	22,18 ± 4,59	14,00	32,70	0,001

BMI: body mass index SD: standard deviation

2.3. Comparison by lifestyle :

- Tobacco :

Our study concluded that 73% of the patient group and 73% of the control group smoked, with no significant difference (p=0.99).

- Alcohol :

Alcohol consumption was 17% in the patient group and 13% in the control group.control with no significant difference (p =0.718).

2.4. Results of the food survey :

2.4.1. Comparison of groups according to eating habits :

- Average water consumption :

Water consumption was low (<1L/d) in 47% of patients and 30% of controls (p=0.791). The other results for the level of water consumption are shownin Figure 22 and there was no statistically significant difference between the groups (p=0.297).

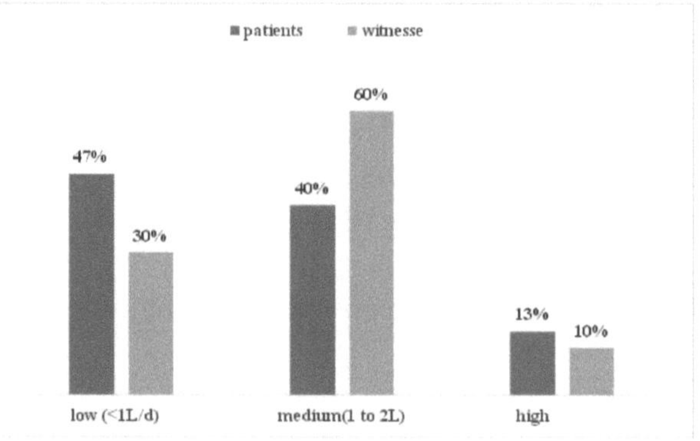

Figure 22: Comparison of groups according to water consumption

- Consumption of salty foods :

Consumption of salty foods was not statistically different between the two groups (p = 0.99), as shown in Figure 23.

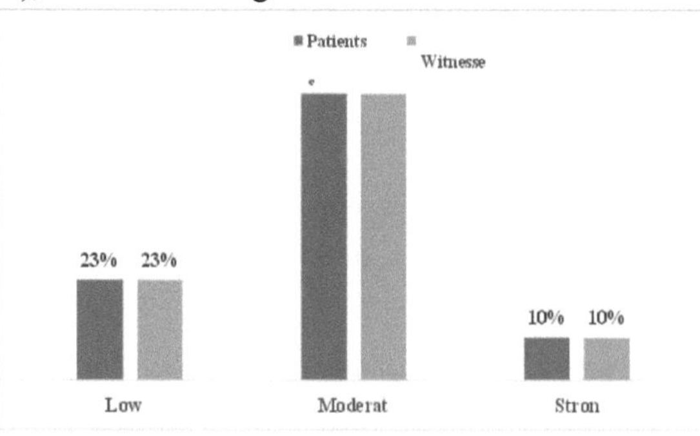

Figure 23: Comparison of groups according to consumption of salty foods

- **Consumption of spicy foods (paprika, pepper, chilli, ginger, etc.):**

Heavy consumption of spicy foods was observed in 43% of patients with haemorrhoidal disease and in only 7% of control subjects. There was a statistically significant difference between the two groups (p = 0.004) (figure 24).

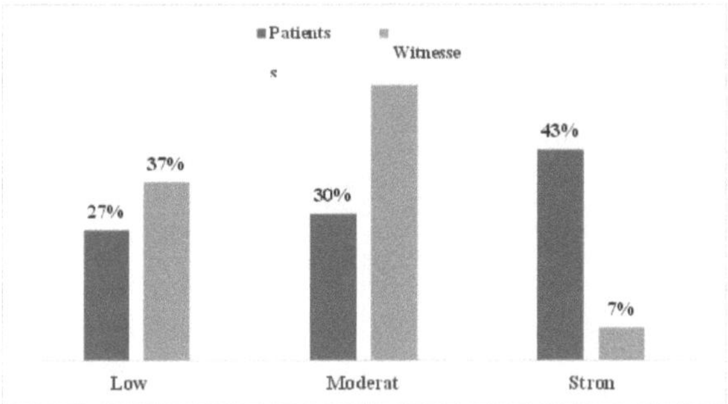

Figure 24: Comparison of groups according to consumption of spicy foods

- Consumption of condiments strong (gherkins vinegar, hot sauces, hot oils, mustard, etc.):

Consumption of strong condiments was low in both groups, with no significant difference (p = 0.892) (Figure 25).

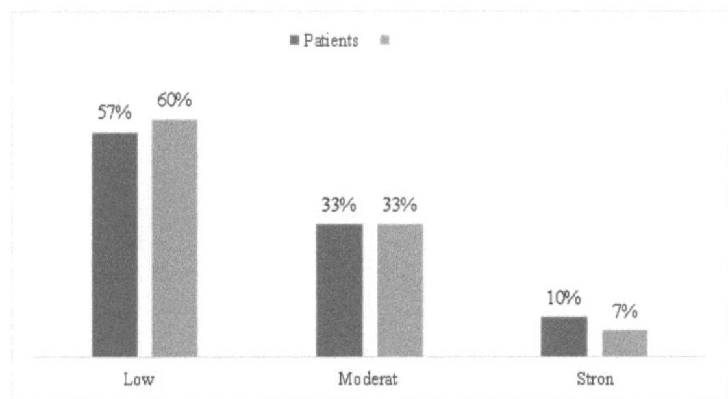

Figure 25: Comparison of groups according to consumption of strong condiments

- **Coffee consumption :**

The majority of patients in both groups consumed just one coffee a day. There was no significant difference between the patient and control groups (p =0.688) (Figure 26).

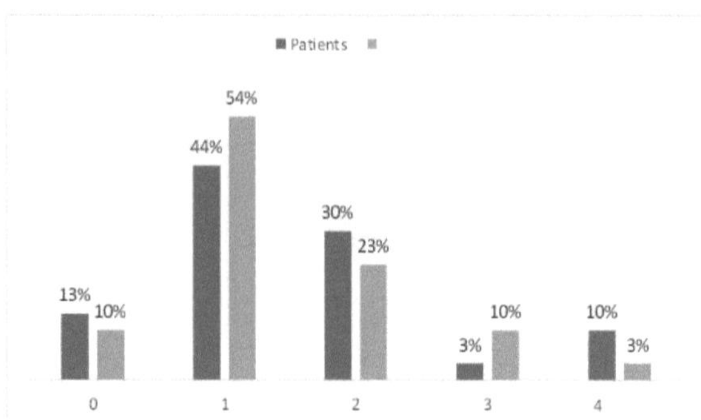

Figure 26: Comparison of groups according to coffee consumption

- **Tea consumption :**

Most patients (60%) and controls (70%) did not drink tea. The difference between the groups was not significant (p =0.417) (Figure 27).

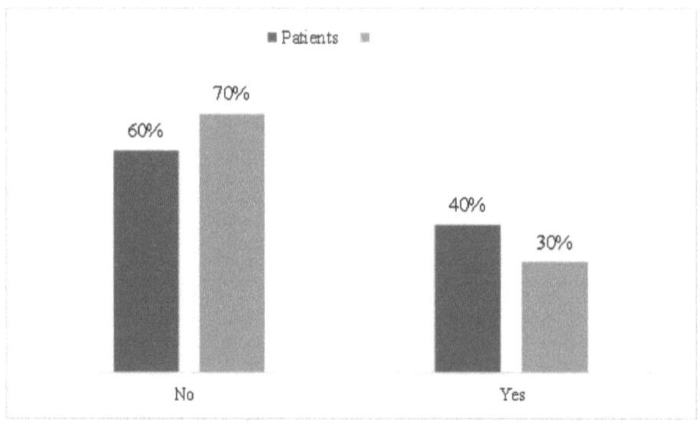

Figure 27: Comparison of groups according to tea consumption

2.4.2. Comparison of groups according to food frequency using the food frequency questionnaire :

The patients were divided into two sub-groups according to how often they ate twice a week. Patients with haemorrhoids were found to eat vegetables and fruit less often than controls, but there was no significant difference. Similarly, the sick group consumed milk and dairy products less frequently than the control group, with a statistically significant difference (p=0.06). However, there was no significant difference between the two groups in the frequency of meat consumption.

Table V compares the two groups according to food frequency.

Table V: Comparison of groups according to food frequency

	Les malades (n = 30)	Les témoins (n = 30)	P
Les fruits			
$\leq$ 2 fois / semaine	37%	30%	0,9
> 2 fois / semaine	63%	70%	
Les légumes			
$\leq$ 2 fois / semaine		63%	0,6
> 2 fois / semaine	73%	37%	
	27%		
Les céréales complètes			
$\leq$ 2 fois / semaine	77%	83%	0,2
> 2 fois / semaine	23%	17%	
Les fruits secs			
$\leq$ 2 fois / semaine	63%	93%	0,02
> 2 fois / semaine	37%	7%	
Les légumineuses			
$\leq$ 2 fois / semaine	94%	92%	1
> 2 fois / semaine	6%	8%	
Viande de bœufs			
$\leq$ 2 fois / semaine	90%	100%	0,07
> 2 fois / semaine	10%	0%	
Viande de moutons			
$\leq$ 2 fois / semaine	98%	87%	0,3
> 2 fois / semaine	2%	13%	
Viande de volailles			
$\leq$ 2 fois / semaine	17%	10%	0,3
> 2 fois / semaine	83%	90%	
Poissons			
$\leq$ 2 fois / semaine	93%	90%	0,894
> 2 fois / semaine	67%	10%	
Les produits laitiers	32%	16%	0,06
$\leq$ 2 fois / semaine	68%	84%	
> 2 fois / semaine			

Comparison of groups at according to of intake macronutrients and fibre: In our work, we found no significant difference between haemorrhoid patients and control subjects with regard to macronutrient and fibre intake. However, calorie, protein and fat intake was higher in patients than in controls. Conversely, fibre intake (g/day) was lower in patients than in controls, with no significant difference (p = 0.406). (Table VI)

Table VI: Comparison of groups according to macronutrient and fibre intake

	Les malades (n = 30)	Les témoins (n = 30)	P
Apport calorique (kcal /j)	1948,87 ± 457,819 [1112-2777]	1918.73 ± 357.691 [1043-2704]	0.088
Apport glucidique			
En %	43.507 ± 4.554	46.367 ± 5.148	0.218
En g/j	214.100 ± 61.579	219.500 ± 51.076	0.965
Apport protidique			
En %	13.583 ± 2.167	12.563 ± 1.788	0.185
En g/j	65.277 ± 14.858	59.077 ± 13.403	0.99
Apport lipidique			
En %	39,483 ± 5,7325	38,183 ± 4,9376	0.482
En g/j	85,347 ± 19,5909	80,730 ± 20,6426	0,478
Apport en fibres (g/j)	19,750 4,9240 [10,6-30,3]	22,017 4,1187 [13,4-31,2]	0.406

2.4.3. Comparison of groups according to eating habits :

- Nibbling:

Nibbling was frequent in patients with haemorrhoids, which was not the case in the control group. However, the difference was not significant (p = 0.3) (Figure 28).

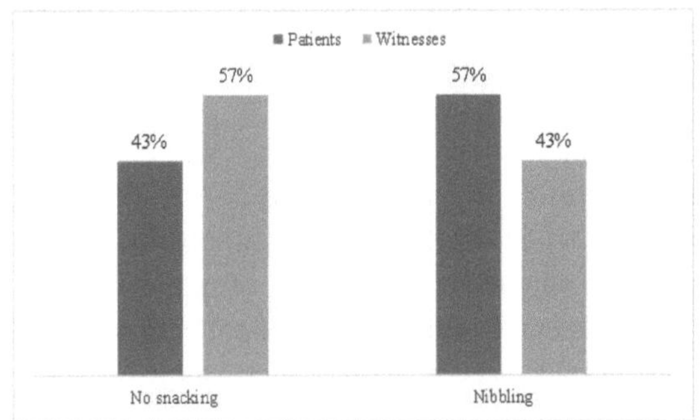

Figure 28: Breakdown of groups by snacking habits

- Skip meals :

Figure 31 shows the frequency of skipping meals in the two groups. not significant between the two categories (p = 0.2) (Figure 29).

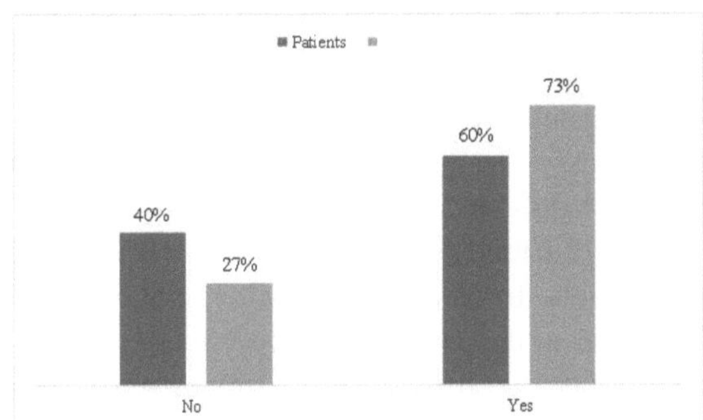

Figure 29: Breakdown of groups by meal size

DISCUSSION

1. Key results :

We conducted a comparative descriptive study to identify the epidemiological, clinical and dietary factors associated with haemorrhoidal disease. To achieve these objectives, we compared two groups of patients followed up in the gastroenterology department of the Charles Nicolle Hospital, one group of 30 people with haemorrhoidal disease and another group of 30 volunteer patients who were being followed up for other pathologies and who did not have haemorrhoidal disease. In our population, internal haemorrhoids were the most common. The majority of cases were grade 2 internal haemorrhoids (67%). In the patient and control groups, there was a clear predominance of females and no significant difference between the groups (p= 0.791). With regard to age, the average age of patients was 46.2 years.± 14.4 years, and was comparable to that of the control group, which was 44.5 ± 19.8 years (p=0.069). Most of the patients were highly educated (37%), married (70%), of average socio-economic status (67%) and from urban areas (93%). Thirteen percent and 7% of patients and controls were obese. The majority of subjects treated for haemorrhoidal disease had chronic constipation (73%), which was significantly more frequent than in the control group (p=0.01). With regard to the level of physical activity, there was no significant difference between the groups (p= 0.518). In fact, the majority of patients had a mild NAP (47%) and 33% were sedentary. In the control group, 37% were sedentary and 33% had a mild NAP. Weight and BMI were significantly higher in the patient group (p = 0.001). Smoking and alcohol consumption were comparable between the 2 groups.As regards the results of the dietary survey, water consumption was lower in the sick group, with no significant difference. There was a significant difference in the consumption of spicy foods (p = 0.004). Spicy foods were consumed more by patients suffering from haemorrhoidal disease. Fruit and vegetables, which were eaten more by controls, and beef were eaten more by patients with haemorrhoidal disease. patients but the difference was not significant between the groups. Calorie intake, protein intake and fat intake were higher in patients, with no significant difference. Fibre intake (g/day) was higher in the controls with no significant difference (p = 0.406).

28

2. The strengths and limitations of the study :

Our study has certain strong points, firstly the use of a frequency survey and a dietary history type survey, which is a specific type of survey. Secondly, the survey data were analysed using Nutrilog software, in order to identify dietary risk factors in relation to the pathology studied. Thirdly, a control group was included to identify factors associated with haemorrhoidal disease. Finally, very few studies have investigated the impact of dietary habits on the risk of developing haemorrhoidal disease. However, there are certain limitations, in particular the small size of the two groups. This was due to the short duration of the placement and the refusal of some patients to complete the questionnaire. The small sample size could reduce the strength of the statistical study.

3. General characteristics :
3.1. The genre:

In our study, women predominated in both the patient group (67%) and the control group (60%), with no significant difference between the groups. This female predominance was found in another Tunisian study conducted by Labidi et al[11]. In this study, the F/H sex ratio was 1.17. However, different results with a male predominance in patients with haemorrhoidswere reported by other studies such as Sangaré(sexratio = 4.5) [12] and Dicko et al (sex ratio = 2.94) [13].

3.2. Age :

The average age of patients was 46.2 ± 14.4 years, with extremes ranging from 21 to 67 years. There was no significant difference between the two groups (p =0.069). These data were close to the results of the study by Labidi et al, in which the mean age of subjects with for haemorrhoidal disease was 42 ± 11.8 years [11]. These findings are consistent with the literature, which has reported that haemorrhoidal disease increases with age, peaking between the ages of 45 and 65, and then decreases [14].

3.3. Education and socio-economic level :

The majority of patients had a higher level of education (37%). In the present survey, educational status had no impact on haemorrhoidal pathology, which is in agreement with the study by Riss et al[15] .With regard to socio-economic level, most patients had an average socio- economic level (67%), 23% had a high level and 10% had a low socio-economic level. On reviewing the literature, other studies have shown an association between haemorrhoidal disease and an increase in socio-economic level [16]. This was not found in our series.

3.4. Personal and family history :

In terms of personal history, diabetes, hypertension and obesity were present in 13%, 27% and 13% of cases respectively. There was no significant difference between groups.In terms of family history, diabetes (60%) and arterial hypertension (47%) were the most frequently identified pathologies. A family history of chronic constipation was noted in 7% of patients. A review of the literature revealed an association between a family history of haemorrhoids and chronic constipation and haemorrhoidal disease [17].

3.5. Gynaecological history :

Haemorrhoidal disease was discovered during pregnancy in 1/3 of the women in our study. Similar findings were reported in the study by Pierre Dalibon et al. The authors showed that during pregnancy, one woman in ten is at risk of haemorrhoidal disease and one woman in five develops this condition after giving birth [18]. On the same subject, another study showed that the prevalence of haemorrhoids generally occurs between the last trimester of pregnancy and the first month after delivery [19]. In line with these findings, the study by Laurent et al showed that thrombosis of external haemorrhoids affected 8% of women during the last trimester of pregnancy and 20% of women immediately after giving birth [20]. Indeed, several studies have concluded that episodes in a woman's genital life such as pregnancy and childbirth are risk factors for haemorrhoidal disease [21,22]. Other studies suggest that fluctuations in the hormonal cycle contribute to haemorrhoidal symptoms [23].

3.6. Level of physical activity :

With regard to physical activity, our study revealed that 33% of patients were sedentary, 47% had mild NAP and 20% had moderate NAP. These results were comparable to those of the control group (p=0.518). The findings of different studies concerning physical activity and haemorrhoidal disease are discordant. The study by Jong Hyun Lee et al, did not find an association between physical activity [24], as was the case in our study. On the other hand, the study by Perry et al showed that a sedentary lifestyle was associated with a high risk of haemorrhoidal pathology [25]. Similarly, the study by François Pigot et al concluded that lack of physical activity is an independent risk factor for haemorrhoidal attacks [26].In the study by Shin et al, it was suggested to continue exercising and to select an appropriate training programme. This helps to maintain a regular system, promote colon health and may even prevent constipation and gastrointestinal problems. In summary, it is recommended that patients engage in moderate physical activity, i.e. 20 to 60 minutes, 3 to 5 days a week, as this improves quality of life and can help manage symptomatic haemorrhoids effectively [27].

3.7.Lifestyle :

With regard to tobacco consumption, our study showed that 73% of patients and 73% of controls smoked. There was no significant difference between the groups. These results are very similar to those reported in the literature, where no correlation was found between smoking and haemorrhoidal disease [24,25]. In contrast, Soo Hong et al, in their study, concluded that smoking was an independent factor in haemorrhoidal disease [28]. Alcohol consumption was highest in the patient group (17%) compared with the control group (13%), with no statistically significant difference (p= 0.718). Data concerning the association between alcohol and haemorrhoidal disease are controversial. Some studies have shown that there is no statistical relationship between alcohol and haemorrhoids [16,25,29,30]. On the other hand, Pigot et al concluded that alcohol consumption is a risk factor for haemorrhoidal attacks [26]. In the same context, a case-control study showed that alcohol is a factor favouring haemorrhoidal pathology (p= 0.01) [6].

4. Anthropometric measurements :

The average weight of patients was 74.6 ± 18.34 kg and the average BMI was 28.99 ± 5.86 kg/m². Overweight, grade 1 obesity and grade 2 obesity were found in 37%, 10% and 7% of patients respectively. Our survey revealed a statistically significant difference in weight and BMI between the two groups (p=0.001). Our results were in line with the literature. For example, the study by Riss et al showed that obesity has a significant impact on the onset of haemorrhoidal disease. In fact, any increase in BMI increased the risk of haemorrhoidal disease by 3.5% [31]. Similarly, other studies have confirmed the correlation between haemorrhoidal disease and obesity [15,24]. However, Peery et al found no correlation between haemorrhoids and overweight or obesity [25].

5. Clinical features :
5.1. Classes of haemorrhoids :

Internal haemorrhoids were the most common in our population (60%) with a predominance of grade 2 internal haemorrhoids (67%). In contrast, in the study by Riss et al, grade 1 internal haemorrhoids were the most common (72.89%) [15]. This could be explained by the operator-dependent nature of the classification of haemorrhoids, particularly the differentiation between grades 1 and 2.

5.2. Transit disorders :

Compared to the control group, chronic constipation was common in patients with haemorrhoidal disease. In fact, 43% had a chronic history of constipation and 73% had constipation at the time of the survey. This transit disorder was significantly more frequent than in the control group (p= 0.01). Chronic constipation is considered an important risk factor for haemorrhoidal disease. This has been demonstrated in our study and in the literature. For example, a study published by Diarra M et al, concluded that constipation was a major risk factor for the onset of haemorrhoids (58.3% of patients suffering from haemorrhoids were constipated)[32] . Similarly, a Saudi study showed that 40% of subjects with haemorrhoids hadreported chronic constipation [17]same context, Peery et al, in their study, concluded that constipation of at least 25% of thetime was associated with an increased prevalence of haemorrhoidal disease [25]. These data were confirmed by Riss et al, who published a cross-sectional study of participants who had undergone colonoscopy, and found that constipation was significantly more frequent in patients with haemorrhoids than in patients without haemorrhoids (P= 0.0113) [31]. This association between haemorrhoidal disease and constipation may be explained by efforts to evacuate hard stools, which may trigger haemorrhoidal pathology and associated signs [33,34]. Rarer studies have shown no association between constipation and haemorrhoidal disease such as the study by Johanson et al [35].As for diarrhoea, no difference was found between the two groups. These findings are inconsistent with the results of previous studies which found a significant association between diarrhoea and the presence of haemorrhoids [21,35,36].

5.3. Other functional signs :

The prevalence of rectal discharge in our study (67%) was higher than that found in the study by Pigot et al (56%)[26]. Higher prevalences of rectal bleeding were reported in other studies such as Pravin et al (96%)[37]. This could be explained by the different grades of haemorrhoids. With regard to the frequency of anal pain, our results were close to the findings of the studies by Diarra et al [32], Pigot et al [26] and Dicko [13]. Our study revealed that the majority of patients (77%), had an effort during defecation, it has been proved by the study of Oberi et al, that the practices of defecation are significantly correlated with a higher frequency of symptoms of haemorrhoids [17].

6. Food survey :
6.1. Average water consumption :

Our survey concluded that half the subjects with haemorrhoids had low water consumption (<1l/d). This consumption was lower than in the control group, but the difference was not significant (p= 0.791). Our results are very similar to those reported in the literature. In fact, several studies have shown that low water consumption is responsible for worsening haemorrhoidal pathology, in particular the study by Sielezneff et al, which found a significant difference between the haemorrhoid group and the control group with regard to water consumption (p=0.008) [6]. Also the Tunisian study by Labidi et al, showed that a daily water intake < 2L significantly increased the risk of internal haemorrhoidal disease [11]. This association between haemorrhoidal disease and water consumption could be explained by the effect of water on stool consistency. It has been suggested that daily water consumption has a significant impact on both the frequency and volume of bowel movements [38]. In addition, the increased water content in the intestine produced softer stools that were easier to evacuate through the gastrointestinal tract [39].

6.2. Consumption of salty foods :

Our study revealed that there was no difference in the consumption of salty foods between the sick group and the control group. We did not find any bibliographical references concerning the consumption of salty foods and haemorrhoidal disease.

6.3. Eating spicy foods :

With regard to the consumption of spicy foods (paprika, pepper, chilli pepper), it was found that 40% of patients and only 7% of controls consumed spicy foods. The difference between the groups was significant (p=0.004). Concordant with our results, several studies have shown that heavy spice consumption is associated with haemorrhoidal disease, notably the study by Pigot et al, which showed that heavy spice consumption was higher in patients than in controls, with a significant difference (p<0.1) [26]. In addition, the study by Sielezneff et al concluded that heavy consumption of spices could be involved in the development of haemorrhoids [6].Contradictory results were reported in the study by Labidi et al. The authors noted that consumption of spicy foods, particularly pepper and chili powder, was significantly less frequent in patients than in controls [11].Evidence has shown that spicy foods have an irritant effect on haemorrhoids, and can also exacerbate haemorrhoidal problems by causing muscle contractions in the gut, which can interfere with the defecation process [40].

6.4. Consumption of strong condiments :

In our study we found no significant difference between the two groups with regard to the consumption of strong condiments (p= 0.892). Unfortunately, we did not find any previous studies that investigated this association.

6.5. Coffee and tea consumption :

Our study concluded that the majority of patients in both groups consumed just one cup of coffee a day, and the difference was not significant (p=0.688). Tea consumption was also comparable between the two groups (p=0.417). Our findings confirm those of the literature, where no correlation was found between the coffee and tea consumption and haemorrhoids [6,11].

6.6. Food frequency survey :

Patients with haemorrhoids were found to consume fibre-rich foods (vegetables, fruit and pulses) less often than controls, contrary to the Consumption of wholegrain cereals and dried fruit was higher in patients than in controls, with a significant difference for dried fruit (p= 0.02). This may be due to the fact that the food frequency questionnaire assesses the frequency of food intake and is not sensitive enough to measure absolute intakes of specific nutrients. Our results are consistent with data from Labidi's study [11], which found that consumption of fibre-rich foods was significantly higher in patients without haemorrhoids. With regard to the consumption of milk and dairy products, we noted a less frequent consumption of these products in patients with haemorrhoids with a difference close to significance (p=0.06), which is consistent with the results of the study by Labidi et al [11]. The latter study showed no impact of meat consumption on haemorrhoidal pathology, which was the case in our study.

6.7.Estimated macronutrient and fibre intake :

When the calorie intake of the two groups was assessed, it was found to be higher in the sick group than in the control group (1948.87 ± 457.819 versus 1918.73 ± 357.691, p=0.08). Similarly, protein and carbohydrate intakes were higher in the sick subjects, but with no significant difference. These results are consistent with previous studies, which found no correlation between calorie, protein and carbohydrate intake and the pathogenesis of haemorrhoidal disease [6,24]. Concerning lipid intake, we did not find a significant difference between the two groups, which is in agreement with the results of the studies by Labidi et al and Lee JH et al [11,24]. Nevertheless, in their study, Seilezneff et al found a higher lipid intake in sick subjects [6].In terms of daily fibre intake, subjects with haemorrhoids consumed less fibre than controls, but we did not find a significant difference between the two groups. Data concerning the relationship between fibre intake and haemorrhoidal disease are still debated. It has long been thought that a low-fibre diet increased the risk of haemorrhoids, but this has not been proven in several papers. Indeed, in our study and in other previous publications, fibre intake was similar between the two groups [6,24,25]. However, in the study by Laabidi et al, the analysis concluded that a daily fibre intake < 12 g significantly increased the risk of internal haemorrhoidal disease [11]. Furthermore, Alonso-Coello et al have shown that supplements of fibre supplements reduced the risk of bleeding by 50% and of persistent symptoms by 47%, but these supplements had no effect on pain or haemorrhoidal prolapse [41]. Given that constipation is linked to fibre intake, recent guidelines recommend dietary fibre supplements as an effective treatment for symptomatic haemorrhoids. In fact, dietary fibre intake is positively correlated with increased stool frequency and volume in constipated patients [42], which could indirectly improve haemorrhoidal disease. A high fibre intake may also soften stools, making them easier to evacuate and reducing the effort required during defecation [43].

THE RECOMMENDATIONS

At the end of our in-depth analysis and with the aim of proposing relevant recommendations to improve the management of haemorrhoidal disease, we suggest the following measures:

- Avoid constipation by increasing daily fibre intake from fruit and vegetables, in order to meet a specific recommendation of at least 25g to 35g per day set by the European Food Safety Authority (EFSA) [44].
- In addition, it is important to recognise the significant impact of the simple act of staying hydrated by drinking water. This practice is recommended because proper hydration by consuming adequate amounts of water and fluids can help to soften stools and prevent constipation.
- As spicy foods are considered a trigger for haemorrhoidal disease in our study, we recommend avoiding spicy foods because of their haemorrhoid-irritating effect.

- Reduce body weight in the case of overweight, given that obesity is the most common form of obesity. significantly a risk factor for the disease studied.

CONCLUSION

Haemorrhoidal disease, a common condition affecting around 40% of the adult population, can affect quality of life despite its benign nature. It is characterised by symptoms such as anal pain, rectal discharge, haemorrhoidal prolapse and itching, and is influenced by a variety of risk factors, including age, hereditary factors, pregnancy, constipation, physical inactivity, alcohol and dietary habits. The primary objective was to identify dietary habits associated with haemorrhoidal disease. The secondary objectives were to identify the epidemiological and clinical factors associated with haemorrhoidal disease. In our study, dietary habits were identified by means of a survey.food history and frequency. A high body mass index (BMI), the presence of constipation and a high intake of spicy foods were found to be significantly associated with haemorrhoidal disease.

BIBLIOGRAPHY

[1] Hemorrhoids Treatment, Symptoms, Causes & Prevention. Clevel Clin n.d. https://my.clevelandclinic.org/health/diseases/15120-hemorrhoids (accessed May 8, 2024).

[2] Montenon I. Haemorrhoids: foods to avoid in the event of a haemorrhoidal attack. Qare n.d. https://www.qare.fr/sante/alimentation-saine/hemorroides-les-aliments-a-eviter/ (accessed May 8, 2024).

[3] Barroyer P. Management of haemorrhoidal disease. Actual Pharm 2022;61:27-8. https://doi.org/10.1016/j.actpha.2022.07.024.

[4] De Marco S, Tiso D. Lifestyle and Risk Factors in Hemorrhoidal Disease. Front Surg 2021;8. https://doi.org/10.3389/fsurg.2021.729166.

[5] Lohsiriwat V. Treatment of hemorrhoids: A coloproctologist's view. World J Gastroenterol WJG 2015;21:9245–52. https://doi.org/10.3748/wjg.v21.i31.9245.

[6] Sielezneff I, Antoine K, Lécuyer J, Saisse J, Thirion X, Sarles JC, et al [Is there a correlation between dietary habits and hemorrhoidal disease?] Presse Medicale Paris Fr 1998;27:513-7.

[7] G J, Kr W. Assessment of the physical activity level with two questions: validation with doubly labeled water. Int J Obes 2005 2008;32. https://doi.org/10.1038/ijo.2008.42.

[8] Classification of obesity and overweight in adults according to body mass index (BMI) or (BMI) n.a. https://www.aly-abbara.com/utilitaires/calcul%20imc/IMC_en_classification.html (accessed May 8, 2024).

[9] Obesity and overweight n.d. https://www.who.int/fr/news-room/fact-sheets/detail/obesity-and- overweight (accessed May 8, 2024).

[10] Fantoli M, Coulom P. Which surgical indications for which haemorrhoids? JFHOD Paris, March 2013. www.fmcgastro. org/wp-content/uploads/ fi le/ppt-2013/pierre- coulommichel-fantoli_ppt.pdf n.d.

[11] Labidi A, Maamouri F, Letaief-Ksontini F, Maghrebi H, Serghini M, Boubaker J. Dietary habits associated with internal hemorrhoidal disease: a case-control study. Tunis Med 2019;97:572-8.

[12] Sangaré D. Study of internal haemorrhoidal pathology at the CHU GT and in the centres d'endoscopie digestive. Thèse Med, Bamako, 2009;94 n.d.

[13] Dicko ML. Study of haemorrhoidal disease in the general surgery department of the CHU Gabriel Touré. Thesis, Med, Bamako, 2007; n°155 n.d.

[14] Frexinos J, Buscail L, Staumont G. In: frexinos, J, Buscail, L, Eds. Hépato gastro-entérologie proctologie 5th edition. Paris: Masson, 2003:395-401. n.d.

[15] Riss S, Weiser FA, Schwameis K, Riss T, Mittlböck M, Steiner G, et al. The prevalence of hemorrhoids in adults. Int J Colorectal Dis 2012;27:215-20. https://doi.org/10.1007/s00384-011-1316-3.

[16] Loder PB, Kamm MA, Nicholls RJ, Phillips RK. Haemorrhoids: pathology, pathophysiology and aetiology. Br J Surg 1994;81:946-54. https://doi.org/10.1002/bjs.1800810707.

[17] Oberi IA, Omar Y, Alfaifi AJ, Ayoub RA, Ajeebi Y, Moafa SH, et al. Prevalence of Hemorrhoids and Their Risk Factors Among the Adult Population in Jazan, Saudi Arabia. Cureus 2023;15:e45919. https://doi.org/10.7759/cureus.45919.

[18] Dalibon P. Haemorrhoidal disease. Actual Pharm 2019;58:46-50. https://doi.org/10.1016/j.actpha.2019.01.019.

[19] Gallo G, Martellucci J, Sturiale A, Clerico G, Milito G, Marino F, et al. Consensus statement of the Italian society of colorectal surgery (SICCR): management and treatment of hemorrhoidal disease. Tech Coloproctology 2020;24:145-64. https://doi.org/10.1007/s10151-020-02149-1.

[20] Abramowitz L, Benabderrhamane D, Philip J, Pospait D, Bonin N, Merrouche M. [Haemorrhoidal disease in pregnancy]. Presse Medicale Paris Fr 1983 2011;40:955-9. https://doi.org/10.1016/j.lpm.2011.06.015.

[21] Denis J. [A study of some etiological factors in hemorroidal disease (author's transl)]. Arch Fr Mal App Dig 1976;65:529-36.

[22] SAINT P, A P. ANUS AND FEMALE GENITAL PATHOLOGY. ANUS Pathol GENITALE Fem 1976.

[23] Parturier-Albot M, Rouzotte P, Elizalde N. [Haemorrhoids and the genital life of the woman (author's transl)]. Arch Fr Mal App Dig 1976;65:537-40.

[24] Lee J-H, Kim H-E, Kang J-H, Shin J-Y, Song Y-M. Factors Associated with Hemorrhoids in Korean Adults: Korean National Health and Nutrition Examination Survey. Korean J Fam Med 2014;35:227. https://doi.org/10.4082/kjfm.2014.35.5.227.

[25] Peery AF, Sandler RS, Galanko JA, Bresalier RS, Figueiredo JC, Ahnen DJ, et al. Risk Factors for Hemorrhoids on Screening Colonoscopy. PLOS ONE 2015;10:e0139100. https://doi.org/10.1371/journal.pone.0139100.

[26] Pigot F, Siproudhis L, Allaert F-A. Risk factors associated with hemorrhoidal symptoms in specialized consultation. Gastroenterol Clin Biol 2005;29:1270-4. https://doi.org/10.1016/s0399-8320(05)82220-1.

[27] Je S, Hk J, Th L, Y J, H L, Kh S, et al. Guidelines for the Diagnosis and Treatment of Chronic Functional Constipation in Korea, 2015 Revised Edition. J Neurogastroenterol Motil 2016;22. https://doi.org/10.5056/jnm15185.

[28] Hong YS, Jung KU, Rampal S, Zhao D, Guallar E, Ryu S, et al. Risk factors for hemorrhoidal disease among healthy young and middle-aged Korean adults. Sci Rep 2022;12:129. https://doi.org/10.1038/s41598-021-03838-z.

[29] Hong J, Kim I, Song J, Ahn BK. Socio-demographic factors and lifestyle associated with symptomatic hemorrhoids: Big data analysis using the National Health insurance Service-National Health screening cohort (NHIS-HEALS) database in Korea. Asian J Surg 2022;45:353-9. https://doi.org/10.1016/j.asjsur.2021.06.020.

[30] Acheson RM. Haemorrhoids in the adult male; a small epidemiological study. Guys Hosp Rep 1960;109:184-95.

[31] Riss S, Weiser FA, Schwameis K, Mittlböck M, Stift A. Haemorrhoids, constipation and faecal incontinence: is there any relationship? Colorectal Dis Off J Assoc Coloproctology G B Irel 2011;13:e227-233. https://doi.org/10.1111/j.1463- 1318.2011.02632.x.

[32] Diarra M, Konaté A, Souckho AÉK, Kassambara Y, Tounkara M, Sangaré D, et al [Internal hemorrhoid disease at the digestive endoscopy center of the Gabriel Toure University Hospital of Bamako]. Mali Med 2015;30:38-41.

[33] SOULLARD J. Do haemorrhoids exist? Rev proct 1981; 1: 32-34. n.d.

[34] SUDUCA P.; SUDUCA JM. Les hémorroïdes. EMC, Edit technique, Paris, Estomac Intestin, 1990, 9086A105 : 12- 20. n.d.

[35] Johanson JF, Sonnenberg A. Constipation is not a risk factor for hemorrhoids: a case- control study of potential etiological agents. Am J Gastroenterol 1994;89:1981-6.

[36] Delcò F, Sonnenberg A. Associations between hemorrhoids and other diagnoses. Dis Colon Rectum 1998;41:1534-41; discussion 1541-1542.https://doi.org/10.1007/BF02237302.

[37] Gupta PJ. Novel approach to advanced hemorrhoidal disease. Romanian J Gastroenterol 2005;14:361-6.

[38] Klauser AG, Beck A, Schindlbeck NE, Müller-Lissner SA. Low fluid intake lowers stool output in healthy male volunteers. Z Gastroenterol 1990;28:606-9.

[39] Anti M, Pignataro G, Armuzzi A, Valenti A, Iascone E, Marmo R, et al. Water supplementation enhances the effect of high-fiber diet on stool frequency and laxative consumption in adult patients with functional constipation.

Hepatogastroenterology 1998;45:727–32.

[40] Ltd HP. Five Food People With Hemorrhoids Should Avoid. HealthMatch 2022. https://healthmatch.io/hemorrhoids/5-foods-to-avoid-with-hemorrhoids (accessed May 13, 2024).

[41] Alonso-Coello P, Mills E, Heels-Ansdell D, López-Yarto M, Zhou Q, Johanson JF, Guyatt G. Fibre for the treatment of haemorrhoid complications: a systematic review and meta-analysis. Suis J Gastroenterol. 2006 n.d.

[42] Spiller RC. Pharmacology of dietary fibre. Pharmacol Ther 1994;62:407-27. https://doi.org/10.1016/0163-7258(94)90052-3.

[43] How to add more fibe to your diet. Mayo Clin n.d. https://www.mayoclinic.org/healthy-lifestyle/nutrition-and-healthy-eating/in-depth/fiber/art-20043983 (accessed May 13, 2024).

[44] EFSA Panel on Dietetic Products, Nutrition, and Allergies (NDA). Scientific Opinion on Dietary Reference Values for carbohydrates and dietary fibre. EFSA J 2010;8:1462. https://doi.org/10.2903/j.efsa.2010.1462.

Appendix 1: Questionnaire

Date:
File no
File no.

1. Identification :

Full name:

Telephone number:

Age

Gender: Male Female

Marital status: Single Married Divorced

Level of education: Primary Secondary   Higher None

Occupation:Student Employee

Self-employed Unemployed Housewife Socio-economic status: Low Medium Good Geographical origin: Urban Rural

Level of physical activity :

Sedentary (little or no exercise)

Light Moderate Active

2. ATCDS :
Personal
Family

Diabetes HTA
Obesity
Chronic constipation Diarrhoea
Digestive disorders
Other Which ones? .
History of pregnancy: No Yes If yes, how many times?

3. Physical examination :

Weight :(Kg)

Height(m)

Waist circumference:(cm)

BMI(Kg/m²)

4. Biological examination :

Haemoglobin:

5. Functional signs :

Constipation: Yes No If yes, since when?

Number of bowel movements per 24 hours:

Effort to defecate: Yes No Anal pain: Yes No

Chest pain:Yes No

Colonoscopy examination: Yes No

Colonoscopy results:

Classification of haemorrhoids :

Internal External For internal haemorrhoids :

Stage 1

Stage 2

Stage 3

Stage 4

Presence of thrombosis: Yes   No

Treatment prescribed:

6. Eating habits :

Smoking:Yes No
Quit date:
If so, how many?
When?
Alcohol: Yes No

Date stopped:

If yes, consumption: Regular Occasional

Average water consumption: <1L 1-2L 2-3L

Consumption of salty foods :

Low Moderate High

Consumption of spicy foods (paprika, pepper, chilli, ginger, horseradish, etc.):

Low Moderate High

Consumption of strong condiments (pickled vegetables, vinegar, hot sauces, hot oils, mustard, etc.):

Low Moderate High Consumption of caffeinated drinks :

Coffee Yes No

If yes, how many times a day?

Tea:Yes No

If yes, how many times a day?

Cooking mode :

Grilling Steaming

Oven

Frying Yes No

If yes:

Sweet Salty Sweet and salty Skip meals:Yes No

Duration of meal :

<10min between 10 and 20 min>20min Mastication:YesNo

Dental condition:

Normal

Poor

Appendix 2: Weekly food consumption frequency questionnaire

Foodstuffs	Frequency of consumption/week
Fruit	
Vegetables	
Wholegrain cereals	
Pulses	
Dried fruit	
Sheep	
Steers	
Poultry	
Fish	
Milk and dairy products	

Appendix 3: Food survey

Meals and timetable	Composition	Frequency/ week
Breakfast à..............		
Morning snack à...................		
Lunch à..................		
Afternoon snack at		
Dinner at		
Evening snack à.................		

Appendix 3: Quantitative assessment of food intake

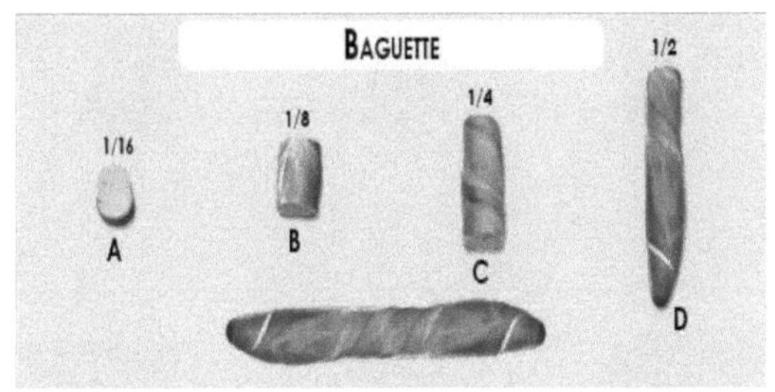

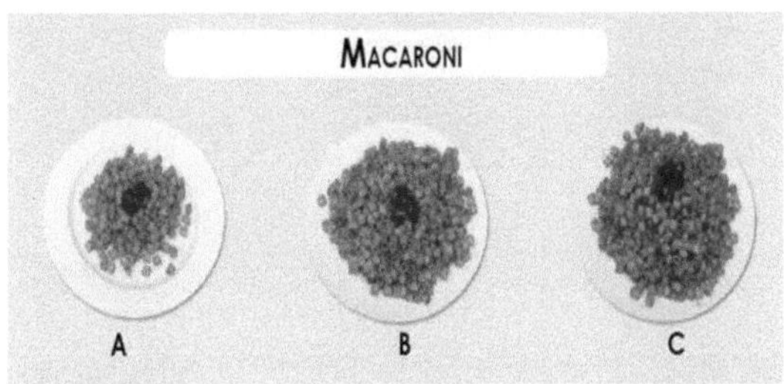

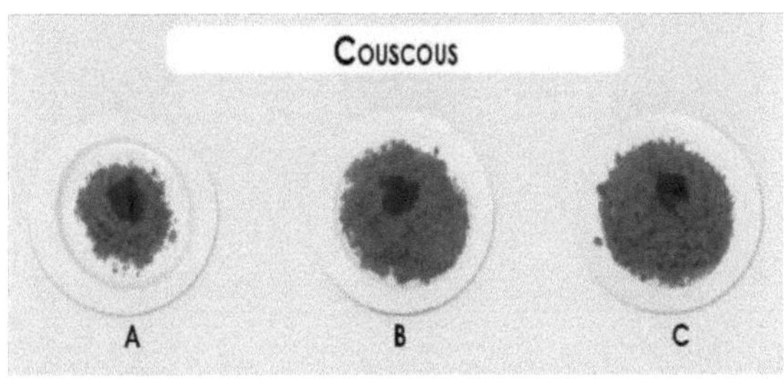

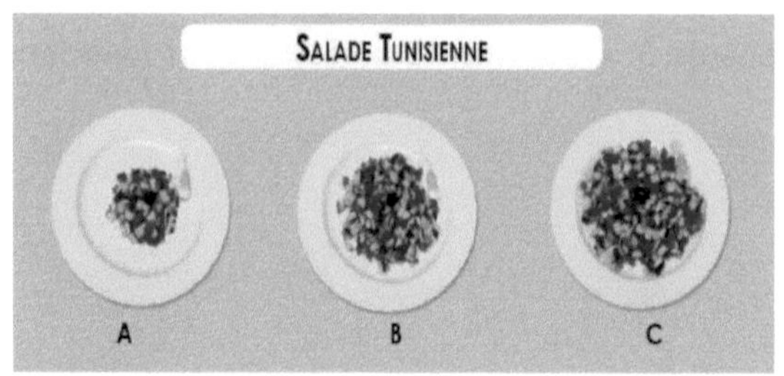
SALADE TUNISIENNE
A
B
C

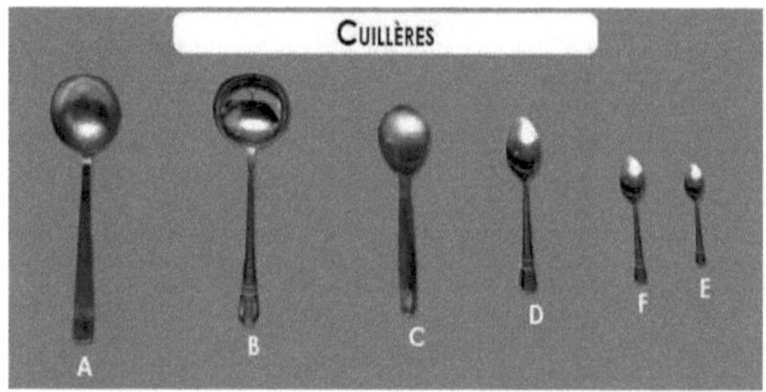
CUILLÈRES
A
B
C
D
F
E

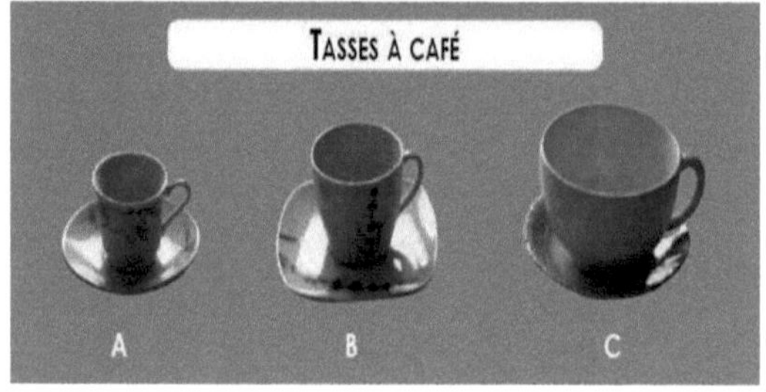
TASSES À CAFÉ
A
B
C

	A	B	C	D	E	F
Baguette	10 gr	32 gr	62 gr	125 g	250 g	
Pasta	100 g	250 g	400 g			
Couscous	100 g	250 g	400 g			
Salad Tunisian	70 gr	140 g	190 g			
Spoons	100 g	60 g	25 gr	10 gr	3gr	2gr
Coffee cups	60 g	100 g	300gr			

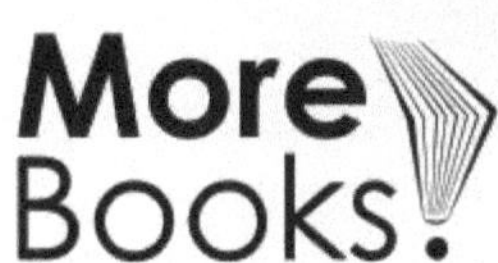

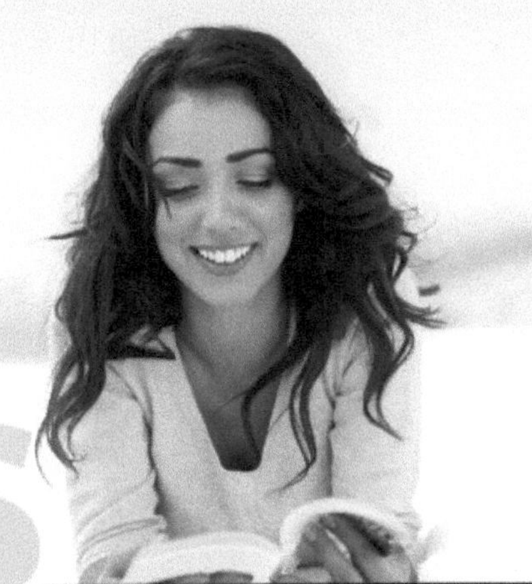

yes
I want morebooks!

Buy your books fast and straightforward online - at one of world's fastest growing online book stores! Environmentally sound due to Print-on-Demand technologies.

Buy your books online at
www.morebooks.shop

Kaufen Sie Ihre Bücher schnell und unkompliziert online – auf einer der am schnellsten wachsenden Buchhandelsplattformen weltweit! Dank Print-On-Demand umwelt- und ressourcenschonend produzi ert.

Bücher schneller online kaufen
www.morebooks.shop

info@omniscriptum.com
www.omniscriptum.com

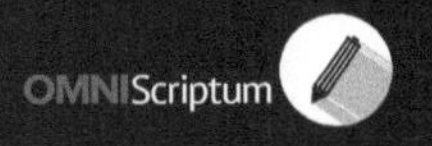

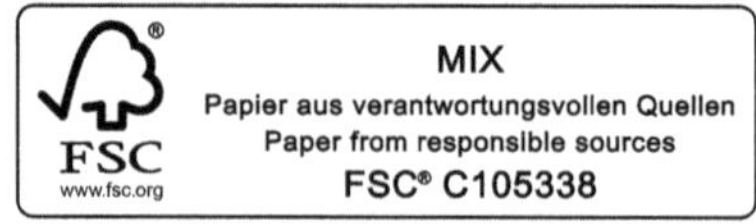

Printed by Books on Demand GmbH, Norderstedt / Germany